HOW TO SOLVE ANY problem!

Meta-Strategies for life!

The Rogue Hypnotist

Also in this internationally bestselling series...

How to Hypnotise Anyone - Confessions of a Rogue Hypnotist.

Now in French: Comment Hypnotiser N'importe qui - Les Confidences d'un Hypnotiseur Rebelle.

Mastering Hypnotic Language - Further Confessions of a Rogue Hypnotist.

Powerful Hypnosis - Revealing Confessions of a Rogue Hypnotist.

Forbidden Hypnotic Secrets! - Incredible confessions of the Rogue Hypnotist.

Wizards Of Trance - Influential confessions of a Rogue Hypnotist.

Crafting Hypnotic Spells! - Casebook confessions of a Rogue Hypnotist.

Hypnotically Deprogramming Addiction - Strategic confessions of a Rogue Hypnotist.

Hypnotically Annihilating Anxiety - Penetrating confessions of a Rogue Hypnotist.

Weirdnosis - Astounding confessions of a Rogue Hypnotist.

The Force of Suggestion part 1: Foundations.

The Force of Suggestion part 2: Changing Perceptions.

The Force of Suggestion part 3: Trojan Horses.

Persuasion Force volume 1: Everyday Psi-Ops.

Persuasion Force volume 2: Alchemical Persuasion.

Persuasion Force volume 3: Invasion of the Mind.

How to Manipulate Everyone - level 1: Exposing the Mind Benders.

How to Manipulate Everyone - level 2: Defend Your Mind!

How to Manipulate Everyone - level 3: Taking Control.

The Confidence Book - How to Stay Sane in a World Gone Mad. Self-help that works series.

How to Block Brainwashing! Manual 1: The Soul Stealers!

How to Block Brainwashing! Manual 2: Downloading Delusions!

How to Block Brainwashing! Manual 3: Selling Hell.

Wicked Teeth - The Secret History of Werewolves (cults/folklore). The Rogue Hypnotist investigates.

Seductive Blood - The Horrific History of Vampires (cults/folklore). The Rogue Hypnotist investigates.

Disclaimer: This book is for entertainment and educational purposes only. The reader is expected to use the information within responsibly. This book is not a substitute for appropriate therapy where required. Any repetition is by design. The unique expression of the material in this book remains the copyright of the Rogue Hypnotist.

FACING REALITY.

A book on problems?

Sure, why not? People want to solve problems of all varieties. But what's the *best way* to solve problems? What things have worked best? Are there patterns of problem solving that are effective, efficient, and reputable? Can we systematise them somehow?

If you had a structure for general problem solving you would have a powerful meta-tool, would you not? That is what this book will give you. Prepare to see problems as a great deal more easy to deal with then you ever did before…

The problem is not problems, which are essential, it's the way we look at them and the ways and means we employ to solve them that might be a problem.

What is a 'meta-strategy'? A strategic way for generating success strategies.

This book is a follow up book to The Confidence Book I wrote. You do not have to have read it to get all you need from this. The first book in this series was surprisingly successful - to me. I think this book too will help…

THE ROGUE WHAT?

We all solve problems every day. Some of us solve specialist types of problems for a while; as I did as a 'professional hypnotherapist'. People came to me with myths called 'mental health problems'. You might as well as call them that as anything else. All were caused by beliefs and behaviours that caused pain, and a failure to solve the real problems my clients faced.

When we're tense it is hard to see the world objectively. Molehills become unscalable mountains. There is also a great myth that tough times bring out 'the best' in people; nope, often it's the worst that that rears its ugly head.

I helped people solve a certain category of problems by using ideas, techniques, sly subterfuge, and a bit of charm. Addiction processes have a positive intent: to make a person feel better. The short-term goal may be met, but it will also be followed by long-term bad consequences. Accept the intent, alter the response.

Problem solving is often clumsy, ill-thought out, and muddled with a lot of people. My hope is that this book will give you a new way to consistently think about problems and solutions so that you get better, quicker, more fulfilling results. Imagine your car has broken down. You need a bunch of people to give you a push to get the engine started. Then you're off to the races again.

I helped a lot of people feel well and whole again. Optimistic that they could face the challenges of life with new vigour and energy. I had a 99.9% success rate, if someone wanted to get 'better'. Do you REALLY want to get better?

I have written multiple internationally bestselling books on NLP, hypnosis, suggestion, persuasion, manipulation, cults, psychopaths and more. All my books are bestsellers. I know how to solve problems, and as a consequence I have lived a really interesting, enriching life. And now, I am going to show you, with a few pointers, how to solve problems much more easily. Ready?

HYPNOSIS AND TRANCE?

You don't have to be hypnotised, or *go into a trance* to get all you need from this book. *Your unconscious* mind can allow you to *enter a gently focused learning state* whenever you need to. Now. Some people let me know that reading a book like this works best in one sitting. I don't know. Each and both of you do. Get comfy - and only take that from this that enhances your efforts most.

If it is minded to, and if it thinks it will help the unconscious can allow you to *experience a deep knowing mood*...

You might notice the words, sounds around you. You might *become totally absorbed* - in this process...New ideas. If your mind wanders that's fine. It means you are clarifying things in a highly personal way. Your attention can come back to these words when you're ready...

We go in and out of trance all day. Light trance, deep trance. Medium trance. You don't need to be entranced at all to get 100% of what you really, deeply need from this book. People mistakenly think a book is the end. It's just the beginning...

Reading a book, watching a great movie, *focusing in* all require a degree of hypnosis...Hypnosis is normal, safe, and natural. But you don't need hypnosis as ideas are quite hypnotic things anyway. Are they not? Ignore anything you disagree with...for this is your experience...

Some people go to sleep and wake up changed. The dreaming mind can do many things that can surprise and delight you!

WANTS AND NEEDS.

We all want something. There are many things that we need. Our wants and needs may interact. We have to have our needs fulfilled otherwise we'll die. Wants are things that would make life more wonderfully satisfying.

When you want anything you set a goal to achieve it. BINGO! This is where we encounter our best friend: THE PROBLEM. The problem is a hurdle standing in our path stopping us easily getting our want. But if there were no problems all the challenge and adventure of life would go out of the window. The fact is problems are the experiences that shape and mould who we are, and who we will become.

Problems are of two varieties: internal or external. Either something 'in us' prevents us achieving our aim or something out there is stopping us. There are only two types of problems, the solvable and the unsolvable. Don't worry about the second variety. Focus on what you can solve. Sometimes a problem is conquered through endurance: you simply outlast or outlive the thing that caused the problem. But that's a passive response. The best thing to do is to work out the best way to *overcome the problem*.

WORD ORIGINS.

By the 14th century the word *probleme* meant a riddle. A difficult question that needed discussion. A scientific subject that required investigation.

The Latin version was *problema*, from the same Greek word which meant - a task, that which is preposed, a question. It also meant a headland, anything that projected, a promontory: AND a fence and barrier. Ah! Now we're getting somewhere. It also meant a problem in geometry. In this sense it meant a thing put forward. From *proballein* - propose. Derived in turn from pro - forward, from the Proto-Indo-European - *per* - forward, by extension, in front of, first, chief, toward, near, against. One variant of this word is ex-per-t. Someone who is good at solving problems in a particular field of human experience. Someone who is experienced and vigilant. The word empirical is another cousin meaning to take a risk.

The *blem* bit of problem is from the word *ballein*, this from PIE *gwele* - to throw, reach, pierce. It many senses this was linked to a concept of pain. Forward throw? A target that causes pain. And something must be done to remove the pain. By an action of some kind that moves YOU forward past that problem and onto the next one AND the next one. Life is about solving problems well. We get stuck and end up in 'therapy' because we cannot solve a problem of some kind. We ask someone to help us. A starving man looks for food, right? Yes, but often the problem is not in you: it's out there. Stop blaming yourself…

All self-help books claim to help you 'how to' solve a particular problem, what they don't do is make you a generalised problem-solving master. After reading this book you will know the meta-structure of all problems, and have a far better chance of solving them.

PST: Problem Solving Tips will pop up again and again as you read and effortlessly integrate the knowledge you need. So let's get started -

PST 1: A problem is usually caused by a specific lack of information, or a failure to take appropriate action to solve the problem.

99% of the time you need a new piece of info and/or you need to act. Effort is involved in problem solving.

WHY DO WE WANT THINGS?

This probably sounds like a totally dumb ass/arse question, but let's have a little think. What makes us really want something?

Needs.

You need air, sleep, companionship, food, sufficient sunshine, water, shelter, money, exercise, challenge etc. You breathe, you take a nap, you make friends, you eat, you go outside, you drink, you go inside, you get a job, you 'work out', you do stimulating things. You take an action to get that thing you need expressed by a verb: drink, eat, fart etc.

Wants.

You want a car. Cars make it easier to get from A to B. You start asking questions: do I have enough money? Screw that, can you even drive yet? How much does petrol cost? Can you fix the car if it breaks down?

PST 2: Identify want - ask multiple questions about how you are going to get that want fulfilled.

Why does asking questions help? It focuses your mind on solutions. Focus on what you want. You want a car to drive: you need money for driving lessons. You need a good instructor. You need to pass your driving test. You need enough money to get a reasonable car of some kind. In other words:

PST 3: You need a doable action plan.

This will be a series of actions that you take. You need:

1. Money for driving lessons: action - get money. Goals require **resources** to achieve. This is the logistics part.
2. You need to select a good driving instructor - look at websites of local instructors. You **seek guidance.**
3. You need to phone/email the instructor that takes your fancy etc. - you *contact a mentor*. This is a common stage in almost all problem solving. More on this later.
4. You reliably turn up and take your driving lessons. You *commit to the change in an active manner.* No problem is ever solved without a degree of commitment.
5. Over a time period the mentor *transfers their knowledge* to you: this may be info or action knowledge, it may be both. You experience a knowledge download. We call this learning.
6. You take the **'test'**: the test is a social ritual that says you can competently join the community of Xers. Those with the skills and knowledge capable of proficiently, perhaps excelling at doing X. By the way you never stop being tested by life. Every day is a test.
7. You save money: often problems require a *present sacrifice* of some kind.
8. You buy the car: BINGO! The problem is solved.

What did we learn?

You need resources, you need skill and knowledge, you need time and commitment. You need to pass a test. You may have to make a sacrifice. So that's it problem solved. We can all go home! On my sweet summer child. If only it were that easy. This is not a 5 page book honey dinkum. We've only just got started. I need to tell you another thing before we wrap up this section...

PST 4: Problem solving should be fun 99% of the time. If it isn't you're probably doing something wrong.

In extremis there are exceptions to this generalisation. We'll get to that.

MOTIVATION.

What's my motivation? The old supposed question of the Method actor. Why do you want X? What will having it, or having experienced Y have done for you that is positive? Focus your mind now on the very many benefits. How will your life be better? Be specific.

Cold-readers and other similar charlatans know that 3 main categories of nominalised (vague process words) experience bother us:

WEALTH - HEALTH - RELATIONSHIPS.

People generally want more money.
People generally want to stay healthy.
People generally want to develop and maintain positive and healthy relationships with others.

There is another category of wants:

SKILLS.

Skills make life easier, in some ways. Most people are trained to be specialists. They may have a great array of actions they can take to solve specialised problems. This is what most training does. However, to succeed at the game of life you need to be a good generalist problem solver; a jack-of-all-trades. When you can analyse any problem and seek answers/methods to solve it well you will be armed with a great advantage that most people don't have.

I am going to teach you the meta-skill of problem solving. I used to solve other people's problems for a living. But teach a man to fish and all that…

INFO.

Most people give no thought to quality of info. You need the best quality info to succeed at anything. Become an info-snob. Only use the highest quality info. As a wine snob only drinks the finest wines etc. A person with the best info wins. 'Intelligence' is info.

PST 5: Good information is a solution all by itself.

Focus on the solution state to motivate youself.

Focus on what you want. If you are motivated by sex, quite shallow, but, we're human, focus your mind on how great that 'sex' will be. That is what motivates you to 'fight'. You focus on the end result. Once you have a motivating goal and an action plan, your powerful unconscious mind will marshal all your forces to help you win. By the way I'm very shallow…

Be of one mind.

Imagine a cart - each corner has a donkey pulling in a different direction. Result? You get f-ing nowhere. To solve any problem you must not be internally conflicted. You can't be a push-me-pull-you. All your inner resources must be in alignment. You must really and with 100% passionate desire want to solve the problem.

If you can do that, you'll solve it.

Inertia vs. Change.

People feel a natural inertia to change. But sometimes you must *make changes*. This requires motivation to change. When this is present all things are possible.

INERTIA - MOTIVATION TO CHANGE
- SUCCESSFUL CHANGE.

Sometimes mere tweaking is required, on other occasions a full-scale psychological revolution must occur.

PST 6: A person 100% motivated and fired up to solve a problem will do so.

Anxiety: your friend.

Anxiety is a signal from your deep mind that shit ain't goin' so well. The feedback from your plans is negative to a greater or lesser degree - you aren't gettin' what you're wantin'. This makes you doubt yourself and leads to a loss of confidence. Once you have effortlessly learnt this problem solving game plan you'll *be far more confident* in general. Anxiety diminishes when what you are doing is working.

PST 7: Pay attention to internal feedback that you're on course.

Problems and focus.

What are you focusing on? When you learn anything in life it demands you focus on some things intently and not others. This is natural hypnosis. Each field has its jargon: esoteric language, and its techniques. The 'how' of problem solving. You need the right language and you need to do the right thing to get what you want. When you start out problem solving, focus solely on that which will ensure you succeed in doing so. Limit your focus to strategies of success. Focus on what works. If you screw up, learn, and focus on doing something that will work next time. There is always another time.

PST 8: You devote/invest energy in what you focus on.

RUN INTO THE AMBUSH.

When most people face a crisis that seemingly comes 'out of the blue' they panic, the want to run away and hide. What you do is **run into the ambush**. When life throws garbage at you - catch it and say: "Challenge accepted!" You are descended from survivors of every outlandish trial known to mankind. You are a problem solver genetically: your entire wiring, physical and psychological, is focused on solving problem. It's your emotion-laden attitudes that screw up the challenge-accepted mechanism.

Running into an ambush is the only way to solve problems. It's a military principle. But it applies to life as things military so often do. For life is one level an ongoing 'struggle' to survive. Soldiers are trained to run into an ambush. Why? One, it's the last thing the ambushers think you'll do. Two, running away allows your enemy to comfortably shoot you in the back. When a challenge faces you *will yourself* to take action to overcome it now. And to keep taking action upon action until the problem is solved. Then you'll face the next one, and on and on.

PST 9: You are a born problem solver - take the problem by the balls!

Face the problem: name the problem.

You cannot overcome a problem you cannot squarely face and name accurately. When faced with a problem ask: what is the specific problem now? Identify it and honestly name it, however painful or jarring using accurate, descriptive language is.

PST 10: Those who cannot name the *real* problem cannot solve it.

Identifying the problem.

Related to the last point, but developed…Many people fail to even begin to solve a problem because they cannot accurately assess what it is. Often this is due to a distortion of perception, previous brainwashing, lying to yourself - consciously or unconsciously, or a lack of info. Lack of info is solved easiest by gathering good info. This also boosts your confidence. With good, helpful info you feel more secure. However, if you cannot admit what the problem actually is, you will never solve the problem. Give up and go home now…

PST 11: What is the actual problem?

The importance of naming operations.

You're still here! Excellent. I knew you looked smart. Military operations have objectives: they are often expressed as 'operation so and so' etc. Name your problem solving actions/plan well. When you do so, you will be half way there. This will energise you. Once you know what is stopping you getting what you want you can take actions to overcome the problem. If you don't want to name it - get the gist of the operational procedure you'll require.

PROBLEM X NEEDS ACTIONS Y = SOLUTION STATE.

PST 12: Name the problem solving operation!

Think in terms of action.

Actors in plays and film think about actions. Not feelings. Feeling come from actions. You do not need the 'right attitude' to solve a problem. You just need to take an action that works. It is surprising how many people persist in doing things that don't work. This can last years, decades, as my therapy practise taught me. *THINK: ACTION, ACTION, ACTION.* Then take the action needed. Now. Do at least one thing every day till you reach your goal. You may need to take multiple actions. Do it.

If you feel tense beforehand don't worry: when you take the right action, you'll calm down, the right action will create the right attitude. Where the body leads the mind follows.

PST 13: Actions solve problems. Actions generate feelings.

How problems arise.

Problems arise due to an unwanted state of affairs - as the perceiver perceives it. These usually exist on an either-or continuum:

Stop - Start: people want to stop an old, unwanted habit etc. People want to start something new.

Improve - worsen: people want to improve their life in some specific or general way, they want to worsen someone else's life.

Keep - get: they want to keep advantages they have, they want to get/acquire new ones.

Create - destroy: they want to invent entirely new ideas/things etc,. They want to destroy existing things etc.

Emotional/attitudinal - thing resources: people want more of a desirable emotional state/beliefs, they want more things.

More - less: they want more of less of some state/thing/resource etc.

Focus/ignore: people want to focus on something or ignore it.

Intake - expel/remove: people want to take in more of something or they want to get rid of it.

Reduce the threat - increase the threat: threats of various kinds are often involved in problem solving. Threats need to be reduced, including de-escalation, or intensification.

Gather - exhaust: you can take in an abundance of resources or use them up.

Produce - parasite: you can create wealth or steal it.

Covert - overt: do you take direct or indirect action? Sometimes deception, or at least cloaking is required.

Freedom - restrict: do you give free reign or do you limit options?

Verify - reject/rebuff: true or not?

Virtue - vice: play fair or cheat?

Defensive - aggressive: do you try to repel or do you 'attack'?

Domineering - submissive/compromise: do you force your demands on reality or take a more cooperative approach.

Conserve - change: stay the same and maintain things or make changes.

Bully - partner: do you 'bully' others or relate to them as mutual partners?

Technical - social: info or human? Is the problem solved by 'technical knowledge' or improved social relations of some kind?

Maybe a bit of both.

These are a number of common meta-continuums. There are more.

PST 14: Ask what is missing!

The 'self-help' paradox.

The problem with most self-help books is that they are written by people who are unqualified to do so. Being famous is not a qualification for anything. Most punters want certain things from self-help novels (I call them novels for most are works of fiction) is help in solving problems of a specific nature. Just because you had a problem doesn't mean you are equipped to teach others how to solve it.

The problem is people believe in magic. They believe there are 'success wizards' who have all the right answers to everything. They believe there are 'magic formulas' and magic spells/words/incantations. All you have to do is go into situation X apply the pre-patterned formula and hey presto! Voila! Everything works out just fine. This is delusional thinking.

Most people seek to solve the following problems:

They want to feel more positive emotions more often. They want to be able to persuade and communicate using magical word formula. They want to like themselves and handle sticky situations. They want their 'potential' untapped. They want to organise their time better than they have done. They want to be 'better organised' in general. They want to have the type of body they desire. They want to know how and what to prioritise. They want the habits/traits/secrets of 'highly successful' personages (twits). They want to stop an addiction process they are trapped in. They want more energy. They want more 'creativity'. They want to stop varying degrees of fear. They want an 'elite mindset'.

They want to 'get over' their childhood. They want almost superhuman mental powers - like the X Men. They want to get rich quick. They want - the impossible! And some people imagine 'hypnosis' will get all this for them. Oh, my sweet summer child!

Many people have bad problems because their goals are stupid leading to further bad problems. I have identified 3 core 'structures' that lead to personal problems:

1. A lack of control.
2. A lack of satisfaction.
3. A general feeling of misery.

Most people make the mistake of thinking *they* are the problem. That there is something fundamentally wrong about them. Incorrect. People imagine a transformation of themselves or their lives will lead to a fairy tale happily-ever-after-land life. You ain't in Kansas any more Toto. You are fine, the problem is you are too scared to be 100% YOU!

PST 15: You are fine just as you are. You are not your problem.

The real secret of 'success'.

I'll tell you the 'secret' to success. If you define it by the standards of the sick culture that currently surrounds us all. Being a psychopath helps. Going to the 'right school' never hurt. Nepotism works wonders. Selling your body or 'soul' will get you marvellous short-term gains. Perhaps you belong to a temporarily favoured group. You think talent plays a part in 'success'? Oh dear. Well, good luck to you darling. For those of us who have brains, sanity, and integrity I offer up the rest of this book to help you.

PST 16: YOU define success on your terms.

Be practical: think practical.

When I was a teenager I had a friend; he was a pipe dreamer. He fantasised about the kind of life he ideally wanted. It was in no way connected to any talents he had. He dreamt of being a successful soccer coach but he couldn't play any sport well. He often told me wistfully of varying pipe dreams he had. To my knowledge he achieved not one.

Another person I knew, an acquaintance, worshipped himself as a young man. In this fantasy his parents willingly indulged him. He was better than everyone at everything - in his mind. He therefore failed to improve at anything. He achieved nothing extraordinary and admitted to a friend of a friend in a pathetic confessional on a London train that he had made all the wrong decisions in life. There is something pitiful about him now.

In order to solve a problem you must realistically assess your ability to solve it. This should not limit you too much for man has travelled into space many times. Goals are reached by making your own luck, focusing on what you want, and doing small practical things every day to get it.

PST 17: Imagine the life you want, align it with your talents and resources, be a realistic optimist. Never delude yourself. TAKE consistent ACTION to make anything happen!

All goals are long-term goals.

You can't focus on the now. It just went, and there it goes, I'm holding onto it! Damn it got away! Now it's the past. Oh, hold on here comes the future! Pause. Now it's the past. Retarded.

Even when you are making a cheese sandwich your mind is

centered on a future state called - eating cheese sandwich. Feeling satisfaction in tummy etc. Eating is part of a long-term strategy known as surviving! If you 'live in the now' and stuff your face with 50 sandwiches, what good could come of it? If you live like 'it's your last day', we'll it isn't, so...

Every goal you set requires you take aim, focus and take actions. These actions should be part of a long-term overall plan that I can only call 'living well'.

My friend told me that he hoped if Vladimir Putin nukes England he has the common decency to tell us at least a couple of days in advance so he can go on a drugs and panties rampage. Joking aside, there is great danger in reckless behaviour as if there is no tomorrow. Sunny Jim? There is a tomorrow. The actions you take now will shape that. So act intelligently, have fun, shape your future well. If you don't take control, who will?

PST 18: Problem solving shapes the future: choose aims wisely.

The pessimist - realist - optimist paradigm.

Pessimists are great at noticing all the problems, at worst they can be paralysed into inaction with a fatalistic attitude. The realist only sticks to reality, assuming he or she knows what that is. The fairy-land optimist takes action and thinks that things turn out well in the end, just, err, because. The air-head optimist is often the most disappointed of the three.

So...they all have good points: let's focus on those. You need to look out for problems, you need to work them out. You need to figure out the best solutions. You need a firm desire that you will solve them in the face of setbacks. Focus on what you want. You need to be 100% realistic as to whether your tactics, strategy, logistics etc. are getting you what you want in a healthy, beneficial way.

Analyse accurately yet positively - be motivated to succeed; focus on success - learn from feedback honestly.

And keep in mind Murphy's Law - anything can go wrong. Make positive plans with Murphy's Law in mind as a backup. Anticipate what could go wrong, have a plan B.

However REAL optimists are happier, and always believe that whatever problems are faced they can all be overcome. Optimism works. Optimism and kidding yourself aren't the same thing. Just saying...

PST 19: Real optimism works.

How do your goals affect others?

Many people have ideas about the things they want, however they don't care much about how what they want affects others or the world. At the far end of this spectrum of disregard exists the psychopath. It simply uses others like pawns in its game. But many non-psychopaths equally use others. Humans are not tools. Other people have their wants, needs, beliefs, attitudes and customs. You must respect this if you ever want to create something of some long-standing worth.

Are you intent on profiteering at the expense of someone's quality of life? Do you want to use someone for your own gratification? Are your wants destructive of something good? There is a moral element in all problem solving. We are moral creatures. Be aware of this.

PST 20: Will your goal make the world a better place? Yes! Go for it!

There are at least 10 ways to solve any problem.

I pulled this number out of my ass/arse. The fact is that most people think you can only take one path to solve problem X. Imagine a box in your path. You have to get past it somehow. Your options? Use mind powers to levitate the box! Back on earth...Push it aside. Dig a tunnel under it. Smash a hole through it. Set it on fire. Blow it up. Turn it into sawdust: it's made of wood by the way. You get the idea. Repeat after me class -

PST 21: There is never only one way to solve a problem.

When you face a problem don't get frustrated *get creative*: we'll get to that.

Analyse the problem to death.

There is a great myth that some people over-think 'things'. I have never seen any evidence of this. The evidence is about 1% of people are thinking at all, let alone sufficiently.

When we are faced with a problem we must often analyse it so thoroughly that we know everything about it. Look for patterns. Predictable structures. Faults. Weak points. Ways things can be improved. You get the idea: know the bastard inside and out. Analysis occurs when we notice all there is about some phenomena. Pick it apart! This analysis will form the foundational structure of our action plan that leads to a solution state. Analysis is taking something apart so well that you can put it back together again better. Analysis is not necessarily the same as criticism. Criticism may play a part in analysis. Destructive criticism should be saved for bastards and bastard organisations etc. Who deserve it.

PST 22: Most solutions are found by constructive analysis.

There are exceptions to this in emergencies when we have to act fast and trust our instincts. We'll get to that.

Identifying the Problem Matrix.

I discovered something I called the Problem Matrix when working with therapy clients. This is the sum total of well-intentioned counterproductive habits that the people that came to see me had. I had to undo the entire matrix to solve the problem.

Let's say the 'presenting problem' is a stop smoking session. But then you discover this person has a public speaking phobia. They are addicted to sugar AND bite their nails. That's the problem matrix: in order to help someone stop smoking you have to take care of all that other stuff too.

So how can we take this general principle and apply it to other problem states? It is not uncommon that a given problem is composed of many sub-problems also. You will have to take care of these supporting structures of the problem state if you are to get to the solution state. You can 'attack' each one at a time. Almost like a game of Ker-Plunk!

1. Identify the Problem Matrix in totality.
2. Break each component part - that is the 'sub-problems' into issues that need addressing.
3. Generate the solutions for each sub-problem.
4. Act on your solution idea.
5. If it works - YAY!
6. If it doesn't work - back to the drawing board etc.
7. Continue until the 'solution state' is reached.

Note: solutions are often just the opposite of the problem - too little money - get more money. Not rocket science.

PST 23: Identify the Problem Matrix - solve each sub-problem individually.

YOU CAN'T KNOW EVERYTHING.

Many people hesitate when they should act. You can never know everything. Situations are never perfect. Sometimes you must act in the most imperfect of situations. Gather as much info as you can to make a good decision and then *do something*. Positive changes occur when you apply pressures onto reality. If you do the same thing - which may be nothing, you can expect nothing in return. Inaction is an action.

PST 24: If you want change DO something!

Know more than your teachers.

Remember Darth Vader's famous line to Obi Wan Kenobi: "When I met you I was but the learner, now I am the master!" There is a truth in this. Many people idolise a mentor, so much so that they remain almost totally incapable of criticising anything they said. They fail to see errors in teaching. They fail to go beyond the teacher and remain a mere acolyte of devotion. An intellectual yes man.

Always aim to surpass your teachers, and for your 'students' to surpass you. This is real progress.

PST 25: Surpass your mentor.

War gaming.

If I do this they'll do that etc. 'War gaming' in general problem solving simply requires that you use your imagination and the known variables to make a series of useful 'what ifs'. If you do X what will Y most likely do? If Y does that, what happens next?

Use the 'magic if' to generate a range of possible future scenarios. This will help in your mental preparation and plan development.

What if, what if, what if…

PST 26: Problem solve by using the magic if.

Lose the battle win the war.

On occasion you may totally screw things up and fail. It happens. Failure occurs due to unfairness, lack of talent, underdeveloped talent, a lack of resources, bigotry, an inability to check all the variables that lead to success etc. Learn from it. Get over the disappointment. Do not wallow. Shit happens. You fucked up. There are nasty people in the world. Never make that mistake again. Focus on the ultimate outcome you desire.

PST 27: If you fail dust yourself off and get back on track.

Avoid pyrrhic victories.

The opposite of the above is winning the battle and losing the war: the pyrrhic victory. If your victory destroys you in the process it ain't worth it. Pyrrhus was a king of Epirus who won a victory against the Romans. It ruined him. Too many of his soldiers had died in battle.

Do not use up all your resources so that you exhaust yourself. Make sure you have reserves. Do not engage in suicide missions.

PST 28: Make sure the consequences of goal achievement 'enrich' and do not deplete or destroy you.

Creativity and problem solving.

Creativity is coming up with ideas and then realising them in reality. Creativity is the KEY to problem solving. Every invention started out as an idea.

The unconscious mind comes up with all your ideas outside of awareness. It's one of the things it is built for. Do not force solutions. They often bubble up while you are doing something else. Wonderfully, creativity is entirely free - it costs nothing.

People are trained that some people are creative and some aren't. This is crap. Everyone is creative. Be creative, solve problems. Don't get stressed or stuck, get creative.

PST 29: Everyone is creative enough to solve the problems they face.

Time and problems.

Time is fleeting. Use it wisely. How much time must you give to solving problem X to get the results you want? How long will you have to maintain an effort? Do you have the resources available during the entire time it takes to get to the solution state? During phases of enacting the solution you may need to take different actions.

TIME + ACTION PLAN + WISE/OPTIMAL

ACTIONS = SOLUTION STATE.

<u>Helpful questions.</u>

How long do you need to achieve X?
How often must you do action Y?
When precisely must you do action Y?
When do I need to stop doing action Y?
When do I need to start doing something else etc.?

PST 30: Solutions occur more easily when you use time wisely.

Making your move at the right time.

Sometimes you wait until the time is right to 'strike'. It's like Goldilocks and the 3 bears - you might need to wait for a sweet spot. If you have a little boat you don't set out during a thunderstorm at sea. Wait till the conditions are calm.

Timing is involved in 'fishing'; you wait till you get a bite, then you reel that sucker in. Doing something in a timely way can save your life and make you rich.

Some people do things better at different times of the day. I hate to jog during the day, I love jogging at night. I am at my most alert between 6 and 9 o'clock PM. I like a long sleep, at least 8 hours. What relation do you and time have? How could you improve it so that your performance is optimised?

PST 31: Sometimes timing is everything.

Jump in and get your hands dirty.

I have come to find that you *learn by doing*. Learning from reading or watching is fine as a warm up, but that's all it is. Get in and get your hands dirty. Will you fuck up? Of course you will. That's part of the fun. Do something. Try something else. What works? What doesn't? Wall flowers dance alone.

PST 32: Get in the dirt and solve that problem!

Be an excellent judge of others.

The most important social skill you will ever need is being a good judge of others. A failure to judge a character correctly will lead to pain. Don't project negative or positive fantasies onto others. Judge people by what they do, not by what they say. Notice what actual qualities they have. Trust your instincts and feelings. Trust is the underlying basis of all good relationships.

People who have convinced themselves they have 'low worth' seek out others who confirm that warped picture of themselves. Demand and expect respect. Anything less is a red line crossed. Why do business with someone who has no respect for you?

It is always better to work with people whose companionships is a joy. Most joy and pain comes from other people. Do not be afraid to ditch someone who does not have your high standards. Expect appropriateness and professionalism in 'business'.

Some people have a 'leopard never changes its spots' attitude; which is true 99% of the time but character is not static. Avoid rigidly static definitions of character. Look for nuances.

PST 33: Problems are solved through sound judgement of others.

Prioritising problems.

Problem stacking. What do we deal with first? Make a list. What is your most urgent, pressing problem? Grade your problems expressed as statements:

Get hair cut.
Go shopping.
Stop farting so much etc.

Which one do you want to solve first? Second? Last? Some people suggest you solve boring need problems first. Get the dull stuff out the way. It depends. You might want to tackle a big problem first when you are fresh. Prioritise problem solving. Urgent first. Arm hanging off? Get this fixed. New pair of socks - whenever!

PST 34: Problem solving demands prioritising.

Cooling off.

Some problems are caused by emotional over-arousal: usually anger, panic, sadness, guilt etc. Get away. Cool off, cry. Get your shit together. Process the emotion. When it's subsided and you are clear-headed again, try again.

PST 35: Problems need a clear head.

Do exercise to get into a problem-solving mindset.

I remember when I was first learning about NLP in the way back when days of the 1990s. I started off with Frogs into Princes one day when I was bored at work during a lunch break. State changes. State dependent learning. Blah! The best way to get yourself into problem solving mode is to de-stress through exercise.

Often we clutter and muddy-up our brain by doing what we have to do. A bout of exercise clears the mind of this 'clutter'. I have no idea why. But it does. The post-exercise clarity state is a refreshed one. Don't over-do it and exhaust yourself. When you have that crystal-clear mindset all problems seem conquerable. You know that feeling you have after a great swim, run, or walk?

PST 36: Exercise clears your head nicely.

The problem of getting attention.

Hey you! Look over here. From a homeless or fake homeless person begging for spare change to the teenage beaut who dresses to get the boys' eye - in order to successfully interact you need attention. How do you get it?

By being 'attractive' in some way. Do you have something someone wants? Do you have what they need? Can you communicate that effectively?

Do you get attention in a way that is respectful of yourself and others? Don't take others for a fool. Forcing yourself on others is unlikely to yield positive results in normal interactions.

Use your creativity to come up with some great ideas to get attention. The answer may be grooming and dress/style. Window dressing. It may be just the right words or pictures. A spectacle, sound or event. An attitude. I don't know. You do.

PST 37: Get attention by being genuinely 'attractive'.

USING TRANCE TO PROBLEM SOLVE: DAYDREAMING.

There has been too much waffle written by NLP types and hypnotists about the power of trance to solve problems. Most of it is nonsense. You cannot daydream yourself out of a nuclear war!

But good ideas that help us solve problems often do occur in natural trance states. When you're going for an uninterrupted walk. In the bath. Whilst doing the washing up. A word from someone else can set off a chain of ideas. If you chill out ideas will just pop into your head that offer a variety of solutions.

Trance and creativity are linked. When you are in a highly focused waking trance: or as we call it in English 'concentrating' you will come up with tons of ideas. Problems can arise from a failure to concentrate or by concentrating on one thing and not another. Avoid overloading your power to concentrate.

I have no idea which dumb-ass came up with the idea of 'brainstorming sessions'. I suspect someone with little creativity. When you are idea gathering let the ideas flow out uncensored. When you have a whole batch of 'em: review and analyse. Find the best. Try 'em out.

IDEAS SPLURGE - REVIEW/ANALYSE - SELECT - EXPERIMENT.

Successful living demands experiment. Sensible, fun

experiments. Keeping a notepad etc. nearby can help. Jot those gems down, don't lose them; they can be like feathers in the wind.

PST 38: Use natural trance to generate solutions and ideas.

Mental rehearsal.

Some self-help scammers would have you believe that visualising is tantamount to doing or achieving. Nope. It can help to go through a task beforehand in your imagination. If only to work out the processes you'll use in problem solving. Of itself visualising is like warming the brain up - it is not an end result. No need for formal trance, try doing it in the shower...First I'll do this, then that etc.

PST 39: Mentally rehearse how you want things to happen. Sometimes.

Asking your 'subconscious' for help.

Your mind-body system are kinda like a space suit you wear on earth. They are made to help you survive and thrive. When you begin to focus on a problem the 'other-than-conscious-processes' are working on it too. Outside of your awareness. You can actually talk to your subconscious in your head - simply ask your subconscious to help you. It will.

PST 40: Your subconscious only wants to help you.

Learn from mistakes, please.

Many people NEVER learn from their mistakes. They make the

same or similar ones over and over again. They fail to take learnings from one field and apply them in another context. Mistakes are there to teach us to do something better/different/wiser in future. Make a deal with yourself to have a 'one mistake learning curve'. Those whose **learning curve** is quick do far better than those who keep banging their heads against a proverbial brick wall. Sometimes this is called 'the long short cut'.

PST 41: Shorten your learning curve, solve problems quicker.

Learn from genuinely successful people.

It is impossible to define 'success' in an objective way because people value differing things. Take successful people to mean those you admire and respect. Being famous without ability is not a worthy achievement. Becoming rich through amorality is meaningless. But there are a whole host of worthy people throughout history that you can mine as role models.

Study their principles. That's the secret. You can often learn a lot by being exposed to them, their writings, film of them talking - if it exists. Their life's works. This will all rub off on you in some magical way.

My nephew loves playing football/soccer. So I bought him Pele's really old book on football. I bought him David Beckham's DVD on crossing the ball/taking free kicks.

He can now actually run around players like Pele, he can bend it like Beckham. Funny that.

PST 42: Learn from people who know their shit and get results.

Core techniques + jargon.

All things are mastered by learning core techniques in any field + the unique jargon developed in that field that expresses those techniques.

Jargon can be used to exclude. It can also be part of a process of 'becoming' part of a profession etc., a part of 'our' language, and so can create a sense of shared understanding and belonging to a new 'fraternity'.

Learn lots of things: have a lot of strings on your bow. You never know when it will come in handy. Skills are logistical resources.

PST 43: Problem solving requires specific techniques.

Use the crisis.

Times of crisis create social fluidity: most people panic. NO! Look for opportunities. I'm not talking about taking advantage of people. I'm talking about finding the best path for you and yours so that you survive and even thrive in a crisis. Think about the situation. What do you need to do to prosper? Do it. Pivot!

PST 44: A crisis is an opportunity.

Wars of attrition.

Relentless action can grind a problem down over time. Extend your timeline regarding goal achievement. Some people want everything yesterday. That is not always possible. Some problems require a long-haul mindset. Wear it down. Take your time. As Shakespeare wrote: 'Whatever wound did ever heal but by degrees?'

PST 44: Sometimes problems take time to grind down.

Your situation is always unique.

Some people think that as long as they have a magic technique that worked in the past it will always work. NOPE! It won't. Situations change. History can be learnt from, but the future is never an exact replica of the past. Each problem requires that you solve it in a contemporary situation. You always have a need to experiment and take intelligent risks to see what actions actually lead you to a solution state. There is no one size-fits all, cookie-cutter formula to life.

PST 45: Each problem is totally unique and requires tailor-made unique solutions.

Improvise, improvise, improvise.

You can't always plan, circumstances may demand you *improvise*. You may be taken by surprise or aback by something. As Bruce Lee said, 'Don't think - feel!' Trust your instincts, keep your head, pay attention to intuitions. Improvisation requires general confidence and a sense of humour. Notice the responses you get. Adjust what you do accordingly. Focus on the ongoing flow of things. There are many times in life when you must wing it or simply make it up as you go along. Trust that your creativity is there for you when you need it.

PST 46: Trust yourself. You can improvise when you need to. Improvising is fun!

EMERGENCY PROBLEMS.

There are times when you have to act fast, now. Many people make the mistake of 'toughing it out'. Though this may be necessary sometimes, often the solution is reaching out. Realising and admitting that you need expert help to fix a problem presently beyond your powers to fix is human. I get by with a little help from my friends.

There is a flip side to this: help others in need. Even a small act of support can have a positive ripple effect. Never underestimate the emboldening feeling of coming to someone's aid to the person who needs assistance. The contagion of psychopathy must end.

PST 47: Emergencies may require experts.

Relationship problems.

Many of our greatest woes and pains are in the heart. Our nearest and dearest, sometimes in name only, can be a big ol' pain in the ass/arse. Fix what can be fixed, sometimes you gotta let people go. There is no golden rule that you have to put up with abuse from someone because you are related.

Then there is the problem of loneliness: find a way to connect. Look out for an opening. Make opportunities to meet others with whom you are likely to have a connection. Join a group. Form a group. Express yourself freely. Share your talents...

The Internet has expanded everyone's ability to connect globally;

that's a good thing. Start interactions positively. If it doesn't work out it's their loss…

PST 48: Make new friends, keep the old, one is silver and the other gold…

Take more intelligent risks not less.

Life moves forward when you plan your successes, anticipate problems, deal with ones that arise, and take calculated risks. Risk is derived from an Italian word which means to 'run into danger'. What it really means now is making a wise gamble. Everything worthwhile requires a bit of a gamble. The future is not 100% certain. Would you rather risk the consequences of doing nothing?

When you take all the variables into consideration you can often determine the outcome in advance. Sometimes you take risks because it is the right thing to do. The consequences of inactivity could be life-threatening.

Gambling addicts are taking the wrong kind of risks. Ones that 99.9% of the time are certain to fail. That's why you take intelligent risks. Size up the situation, make your move. Commit. Dare to risk, no risk - no solution. The adventure in life often comes from taking sensible risks. Avoid recklessness.

PST 49: Risk takers are problem solvers.

Make alliances.

Like-minded people can help each other out. From ancient times people have banded together to solve problems - we helped each other hunt, we helped each other build a hut, we fought off aggressive tribes, we pass on our wisdom to the young.

When you make strong alliances based on shared values you will move mountains no matter by how much you be outnumbered or 'outgunned'. It is a vigorous and determined minority that stick fast together that ever have shaped history.

PST 50: We few, we happy few, we band of brothers!

Be energetic to get more energy.

Stress can rob you of energy. Find time to chill out and have fun. This is even more important in stressful times. Having a sense of humour in dark times will energise you. By the way, the way you get more energy is to DO MORE. When you do things you get energy. You need energy to solve problems. Don't drink too much booze it makes you sluggish and robs you of energy. You need your wits to solve problems. Eat well, preferably organic - stay away from fast food. Eat it as a treat every now and again; it has no nutritional value. You can make home-made versions of your fav fast food that can be 100 times better! Perfect the science of the home-made burger! Good nutrition = energy. Exercise = energy.

Beware of becoming a 'carbivore' - eat carbs they give you energy, but make sure you are eating fresh vegetables every day. Too much sun can sap your energy. Drink fresh, good quality water. Don't do drugs if you want consistent energy. Your body wants to give you energy - don't get in its way. When you have energy ALL problems seem solvable. Make sure you *feel energetic* when you go about your problem solving.

PST 51: With your tank full anything is possible!

Highest quality information - 2.

No problem solving is possible without high quality info. Just as the best food is good for you, so too is the best information. This requires sources that are consistently accurate and make your life better as a result. Seek out good sources of info. 99.% of your problem solving will be taken care of. Get good advice. Advice that proves itself useful. Ditch the rest. Most people are lazy info-slobs who expect to be fed info like a baby. Nope! Go out and actively look for it.

PST 52: High quality info = success.

Beliefs that stop and aid problem solving.

Your attitudes are your greatest resource in problem solving. An 'I can't x...' frame of mind will get you nowhere. If you take on the following 2 statements as a credo, and utilise the questions you will build a problem solving frame of mind:

I can solve X.
I will solve X.
How will I solve X best?
What's the easiest way to solve X?
How will I know I've solved X in sensory based terms? (What you'll see, hear, taste, touch etc.)
Who will benefit?
Who will lose out?
What will I gain?
What specific steps must I take to solve X?
Who do I need to influence to solve this?
Where is this problem's weak spot?

The next sentences = problem solving beliefs. Just say them to yourself as if you mean it when faced with a difficulty: you could think it in a determined way, a laid back way, a laughing way...

I am a brilliant problem solver.

I solve problems easily.
I am determined.
I quickly learn from mistakes and feedback and adjust course.
I'm confident I'll find a way.
My creativity creates solutions.
I have smart ideas.
I can learn anything I need to.
Problems are opportunities.
Problems help me learn, mature, and progress.
The is no problem that I cannot solve.
The more problems I solve the more confident I get.
I like solving problems.
Challenges are fun.
All problems turn out smaller than I once imagined.
I am smart enough to solve this.
Obstacles are there to be overcome.
I succeed.
I know how to handle different types of people.
I am good at influencing people.

Repeat these tropes in your head. Soon it will become second nature. Write your own positive statements down if you like. Those above are just training wheels. Say it, mean it, do it.

PST 53: With the right attitude problems are inevitably solved.

Tell everyone?

Some self-help-guru-type-thingamajigs say you should tell everyone else your goals and this will motivate you to live up to your declaration of 'goal intent', or whatever... You can do that. It's far better to just do it, and tell everyone else after you're successful. If you're the type that keeps telling others you are going to do this and that and don't, everyone will think you're a flake and a bullshitter. Anyone can talk a good plan. Do it.

PST 54: Walk the walk.

Most people are robots.

Since most people are highly programmable you should expect them to behave in predictably-patterned ways. When you know the programming they've received you'll know which buttons to press. Which doors to open. Which ones to walk away from. Which ones are hard nuts to crack. Which ones aren't worth the cracking. Find a way in...

PST 55: Knowing their programming = successful influence.

Talk tough do nothing.

Many people talk tough but sit on their bottoms and do absolutely nothing. That kind of person solves one problem for a while: they hide their true character. But their inaction will reveal them for what they are in time. Work with doers who deliver.

PST 56: Problem solvers deliver the goods.

Only associate with good people.

Hanging around with losers and arseholes/assholes is a problem you can do without. Dump them. Only have good, supportive people around you. Half the tension that stops you solving things will evaporate as if by magic. Don't believe me. Try it. Have high standards - why do we demand our food be right in a restaurant but we'll eat any shit from a person? Don't do that! You deserve more.

PST 57: Create a human atmosphere that says YES!

Be kind but...

Sometimes you gotta kick butt. Not violence, necessarily. If someone acts in a shitty way - you gonna take shit or shit right back ten times harder? There are different ways to shit. But sometimes - shit you must. Don't do anything that will get you in legal trouble obviously. You ever penned a really good letter that got results? You ever told someone a home truth? You ever stopped a 'fight'? You ever reminded someone they have a conscience? There's is thankfully more than one way to shit. And you are no one's toilet.

PST 58: Stop shit in its tracks.

What resources do you have now?

Internal and external resources. Emotions, beliefs, ideas, experience, skills. THINGS. Tools. People. Places. What resources do you have that will help you overcome that problem? Which will you need? You have one this and two thats - get the other stuff. This really ain't rocket science. There is a time and place to get basic and methodical. You'd be surprised what you already have in you if you gave yourself a chance. Do you *believe in you*? If you don't - who will? You need to cross a river. You could get a boat. You could build a bridge. You could...

PST 59: Gather resources that aid your problem solving potential.

Retention and regurgitation isn't enough.

Lots of people retain info. They can regurgitate it real good. You're supposed to think about it. Change it. Add - subtract. Improve, develop, dis-card. You are a human not a parrot. What you think matters. Sometimes you let the chips fall where they may.

PST 60: Info is there for you to improve upon. Info serves man, not the other way around.

States of tension - relaxation/rest.

Balance! Bit of action. Chill. Don't burn out. Don't rest too long = BORED! Bit of this, bit of that. Excitement. Come down. Interesting - basic. Wants - needs. Pig out - eat healthy. Rollerblading - gentle stroll with that oh so nice summer breeze. Life is good.

PST 61: Work-life balance or something.

Emotional problems.

There was a great British comedian Tommy Cooper. He had a routine:

Man goes to the doctor and says 'It hurts when I do that.'

Doctor says, 'Well don't do that.'

Many emotional problems are caused by triggers. Triggers + a background of elevated stress = PROBLEM. Is it a thing you eat? Is it a person you meet? Is it a situation? Whatever the trigger is - cut it out. Walks in nature and exercise help. Organic food. Spending more time with people who genuinely like you. Stroke your cat or dog. Play with your kids - magic! Have more fun. Watch a comedy film or show. Take it easy. Go to the seaside. Treat yourself. Triggers aggravate less when background stress is low.

Don't let dumb thoughts become a trigger. You'd be surprised at the shit we say to ourselves that winds us up/annoys us and does no favours.

PST 62: Don't make life harder than it already is.

Problem holidays/vacations.

Just fuck it some times! Take a break from it all. Go off - take the fam, go off alone, go with friends, whoever. Just get away from it all and recharge your batteries. Pretend to be ill and take a few days off work. Nervous breakdowns occur when people run out of energy.

Get drunk, eat too much, lay by the pool, slob it out on the beach. Play computer games. Behave somewhat irresponsibly. Sometimes the best way to get a new perspective on something is to get out of the situation that caused it in the first place. When *you are more relaxed* and in an objective mindset the solutions will present themselves. Don't force it. Let subconscious cooking occur.

PST 63: Sometimes you get away from the problem to solve it.

Focusing on the self too much.

Some people talk about themselves endlessly. This over focus on the self can lead to hypochondria. Focus on others. Talk about, think about the big things of the world - get away from you for a bit. Trivia atrophies the mind. Do something for someone else without wanting a reward. You are important and so is everyone else. There is more to life than just you. Self focus can inflate problems to oversized things. Read biographies of interesting people.

PST 64: Broaden your mind and interests.

PROBLEMS AND INDEPENDENCE.

A degree of independence helps in problem solving. Financial independence never hurt anyone. Resource independence helps. How can you cut out as many 'middle men' as you can? Bake your own bread. Brew your own beer. *Self reliance*. Remember that?

Are you so dependent on others goodwill that you cannot solve that problem? Will solving that problem lose you your job? Are you dependent on someone's okaying your measures for problem solving? And does that impede your problem solving ability? You know what you have to do. Nothing, almost nothing, pains us more than losing our integrity for a lousy buck.

PST 65: The more fully independent you are the easier it is to solve problems.

Attracting with the 'promise'.

Promise = experience, skills, 'attractiveness'.

Every human transaction of worth starts with the promise of something better. Your experiences and skills will attract others to want you to share them with them. You are most attractive when you are fully and freely you. Compare yourself favourably to others. Dress nice. Brush your teeth. Wipe your ass/arse. When you look good you feel good. Make eye contact. People are attracted to people who make the best of themselves. You'll stand out. It says you care. What promises do you radiate?

PST 66: It is promises kept that help solve problems.

How will you know you've succeeded?

What do you want? Have you really, really thought about it? Is it that car? Will that make you happy? Really? Yes, go for it. You really want to go to that school? You really want to date that person? What will having that shirt do for you? What will your garden look like when it's just how you wanted it?

How will that birthday cake look? What hairstyle would best suit you? For now anyway. If you're bald - could your head be shinier? What does becoming better at X mean for you?

What will you see, hear, feel, think, whatever when you have X and that problem is solved? Send out vague - get back vague. Details darling, the details…

PST 67: Want things worth wanting, be as specific as possible about what you want.

Blindness in analysis.

Once upon a time there was a man or was it a woman, who knew everything. They were never wrong. But they had a problem they didn't know about. They could not see the colour purple. They didn't see it because they believed there was no such thing as purple.

One day a purple people eater took a great big shit on their know-it-all head. Their friend asked, "Didn't you see that purple people eater was going to take a shit on you?" To which know-it-all replied - "What shit?" And then the smell hit them...

A note on wealth and blindness: there is something I have come to call 'wealth blindness'. There is nothing wrong with being wealthy. I wish more people were so. But wealthy people often miss things that are affecting other people because their money protects them. If you are wealthy make sure you accurately know what is going on across wider society.

PST 68: Just because you don't or do believe don't make it so.

Communication problems.

Get them to talk about themselves. Only make genuine compliments. The Dale Carnegie classic tips.

Actually listen to people. Understand them and their needs. Most people don't listen to what others are actually saying - they talk over them and only care about what they're saying. Or they're inside their heads practising what they're about to say. So - listen! Almost everyone feels misunderstood. Try to understand.

Women are much better at making suggestions than men. Take photography - male photographers sometimes bark at models. Stand here! Shift out your hip! Put your hand on your whatever! Cool it Sargent!

Women photographers will use phrases like:

*Can we try it with...Let's try it like this...*etc. Not orders - let's try X. Do you know how smart this is? It takes all the pressure off of the other person because you are just trying stuff.

*Actually...*Instead of saying - YOU'RE WRONG! You could say, 'Actually I heard/read/saw etc.' You can use words like 'actually' as softeners. Everyone barks at everyone. Chill.

Avoid egotism - I am right you are wrong. Stick to the facts, let facts be the star.

Listing nouns is not an argument. Making unsubstantiated generalisations/statements is not an argument. Certain people need to know how to talk in a civilised way without shouting. Certain people need to realise not everyone believes the same stuff. Civil debate can be a good thing.

'How do we know this?' This is a good thing to ask if you want to pinpoint a source. It doesn't accuse someone of being stupid or whatever. It is a good way to make someone think about the source of their info, making them aware of where exactly an idea came from. A conversation doesn't have to be a smart-arsed competition.

Calming down a stressed person 101: I once phoned a clothes retailer to arrange a return of goods, whatever it was was too small I think, anyway…

The young woman on the other end of the line was so stressed. Clearly people had been shouting at her, complaining about stuff and blaming her for her company's shortcomings or their own shortness of temper. She was speaking really fast. She was suffering from sensory overload frazzle.

So I thought I would do my good deed for the day. I spoke in a really calm voice. I slowed my voice right…down. I was pleasant and polite. Within about 30 seconds of doing this she calmed down. Her voice slowed down. I could tell she felt better.

One: don't shoot the messenger. Two: treat people as you would like to be treated. Unless they're an asshole. We'll get to that.

PST 69: Communication excellence = problem solved.

Theories of solution.

What works is the solution. For years people believed in Egos and Ids. Inner childs and anal phases. No one got better.

Is 'your' theory the problem in your problem solving efforts. You might need to take that old donkey off your back. Maybe make up your own theories.

PST 70: If the theory is the problem you got a problem.

Problems of injustice.

Injustice of all sorts is a major cause of stress; kids know when things ain't fair. The psychopathic types create unfairness and call it fair. Call them out. Don't stop till the unfair is replaced with the fair. Delusions do not entitle you to a special type of treatment.

PST 71: Injustice is a problem that must be solved.

Seeing problems coming a mile off.

People say you cannot predict the future. This is incorrect. You cannot know everything about the future, you cannot see into the far future. But based on past trends you can extrapolate that they will or will not continue into the future if variables remain constant. The sun will rise tomorrow.

Some problems are obviously looming on the horizon, but many people do not want to face them. The person who keeps their eyes peeled and is prepared will solve problems a helluva lot easier than the person who tries to wing and a prayer their way through life. Being buffeted from crisis to crisis like that ball in a pinball machine.

FACE REALITY - PREPARE - OVERCOME.

PST 72: Anticipating obvious problems cuts them down to size.

Don't create a problem.

Many people create problems. Politicians do this all the time. Avoid looking for trouble; if you go looking, trust me, you will find it. Life is quite tough enough without manufacturing problems that could have been avoided with some thought.

PST 73: If you look for trouble you'll find it.

Looking out for trouble.

I can see trouble coming a mile off. I go into a bar, within 30 seconds I now all the troublemakers. I know which places are out of bounds. I can see political storms brewing. Know when 'economists' are just making shit up again. Create a part of you that looks out for trouble. You'll end up with less bruises.

PST 74: You have a part of you that looks out for trouble-makers. Listen to it.

The resource of DETERMINATION.

Some problems are solved over a long period of time. If your butt itches you can just scratch it. But if you have greater ambitions this will take time to achieve; determination is required. If you want to collect stamps - knock yourself out! You wanna go to the moon? Determination is prolonged motivation until the goal is attained. If you want something badly enough you will be surprised by how much motivation you can access. The determined person will always overcome a solvable problem. Determination actually means no limits.

PST 75: The king of resources in problem solving is determination.

The solution might not exist yet and you may not have found it.

Annoyingly it is a fact that some solutions require outside help to bring about. We search for a solution, try many things, none work. Sometimes a new solution has to be invented. You might have to wait for this. Or you may simply have to carry out a more prolonged search. Persist - times change. Inventors invent. Scientists do better science - sometimes.

PST 76: Sometimes problems are solved with something brand new. This can take time to emerge.

TOOLS - THE 'TRANSFORMATIVE'.

Tools transform things. Many problems need a tool - a method, a machine, an instrument, a way of seeing things. I have a film studio called Maya. I can create feature films with it. In the past people like me could not own a film studio. Now I do.

The computer tool allows access to data beyond imagining. What tools will you need to solve that problem? What is a tool?

PST 77: Do you need a specific tool to solve that problem? Get it!

Aggressive problem solving.

When various psychopaths made their move in the 1980s the book Sun Tzu's Art of War became a very popular pop-psychology purchase. It is true that learning principles of warfare can help in problem solving. Not literally but as figurative, across-the-board strategies. Reading such books can train you in 'strategic thinking'.

The 12 principles of winning a 'war'.

There are 10 basic principles to winning any 'war'. These are no longer taught in the US military. This is my adapted version - the

12 principles.

1. **Objective:** this must be fully definable. Resources are allocated to achieving it. It is fully realisable and obtainable? If it isn't don't bother - for now.
2. **Offensive:** you must seize the initiative. You take actions proactively, you do not react. You control your opponent's reactions by deciding when and where action is taken. This throws your opponent off balance. You control what they react to. Note: defensive wars NEVER work. You must attack.
3. **Mass:** concentrate your resources at the decisive point in space-time. Massive applied force and 'violence of action'. In problem solving I would call this the *overwhelming force of action.*
4. **Economy of force:** allocate the least resources to the least important thing - prioritise.
5. **Manoeuvrability:** aim to place your enemy at a disadvantage. Apply calculated pressure to reduce his sphere of influence. Set a trap. Lure them in.
6. **Unity of command:** all efforts are governed under one command. Committees lose. This is why all feminised societies in history have been crushed.
7. **Security:** never let your enemy gain an advantage. Never let them feel secure.
8. **Surprise:** strike when your enemy is unprepared.
9. **Simplicity:** make everything simple and clear. Complicated = failure. KISS - Keep It Simple Stupid.
10. **Morale:** 'Holy wars' win. The cause is just.
11. **Plan but change the plan:** plans encounter reality - plans collapse on testing - ongoing replanning and reconfiguring is normal. Be flexible in the face of feedback. Constantly update and adjust.
12. **Cohesion:** all struggle is won by collective unified effort. The higher the degree of difference the less cohesion there is.

There are other lesser principles to consider:

1. **Never hesitate:** the more aggressive you are from the get go the

more likely success is. You minimise damage to yourself this way.
2. *Look for signs of weakness:* this is often looked for in submissive, cringing language cues. Kick them when they are down.
3. *Ad hoc fails:* arbitrary tactics fail. Have a good plan, stick to it, apply it determinedly.
4. *Never surrender:* self-explanatory.

PST 78: The principles of war apply to the struggles of daily life.

Taking charge.

Sometimes in life we have to take charge of the situation. Someone has to lead. Someone has to take command. You have it in you to do this. This is not about being bossy. Sometimes it is simply required to herd the stupid. You can take charge by asking the right people questions.

PST 79: There will be times when you must take command. Do it.

The problem of being believed.

Even in the face of overwhelming evidence some people cannot believe in facts. The problem of being believed can be found in the scientist who comes up with the ground-breaking and new and is scoffed at.

As brainwashing is the norm do not waste effort on those trapped in the prison between their ears. Note it, move on, find those with ears to hear.

Let me tell you a true and sad tale. I have a friend who had a girlfriend. She brainwashed herself that she had 'hereditary' Alzheimer's and would die young as her sister and mom/mum had. In her mid 30s she started showing 'symptoms'. Bang on cue. She was hospitalised, put on powerful drugs. She was going to die young. 5 years later she is still dying.

PST 80: Sometimes the problem is that you can't get someone to believe you. Often this ends up being THEIR problem.

To take advice?

The thing about advise is who to get it from. It could be from a best friend. It could be from a stranger, a book. Once you've got that advice you need - have a good old think about it. No matter what the advice is it ultimately is YOUR decision. Advice regarding action without accountability is easy. Ponder - decide.

PST 81: All decisions must be yours.

Reaching out for help - 3.

If you get stuck reach out for expert help. Find someone whose style you like. Find someone's whose expertise leads to becoming unstuck. Never be afraid to ask for help. Beware of creeps.

PST 82: Seek help from those that you get a good feeling about.

Bad hair days.

You ever have one of those days when all your good ideas fuck up royally? Everything goes wrong. You merely wish for the day to be over. Just get through it. Accept this will happen now and again. Vow not to repeat the same mistakes. Learn. Laugh about it months or years later, when you've forgotten the true nightmare. It's just one of those days.

PST 83: Everyone has a bad hair day.

Problems of ignorance.

A great many problems in life are caused by being ignorant. A lot of ignorant people are smart. There's nothing wrong with their brain. They ignore facts: they are an ignore-ant.

To get smart and make the best decisions you need facts: only facts help you solve problems. You must face facts, you must use facts. Leave fantasy for the looney-tunes.

The working classes need to read more books. The middle classes need to stop reading the wrong books.

PST 84: Get informed. You ignore facts at your peril.

Money + problems.

In the world as it is currently configured you need money. Money is an energy. It allows things to happen. It opens doors. Money is a valuable resource in solving lots of problems in a 'civilised' society.

We often need to use money to fix problems. To buy 'tools' or a 'fixer' themselves. Lots of people waste money buying garbage, or they have insufficiently researched the best buys. Do thorough research before buying anything important. These are investments in the widest sense. Vow not to waste a penny of money. It don't grow on trees folks. Look for bargains.

Can you turn a talent, hobby/interest, an interesting life into cash? Can you monetise specialist info? You can diversify your 'portfolio' in more ways than one. If you want/need more money you must priotise that desire.

PST 85: Face the reality that money helps in problem solving.

Trust.

A great many problems in life are caused by misplaced trust. Not only in cases of psychopathic con-ology (the science of conning people), but by putting undeserved faith in persons and institutions that frame themselves as trustworthy without question. Trust is earnt based on evidence-based outcomes/past performance not by an imagined halo.

Misplaced trust can get you injured or killed. Think.

PST 86: Trust develops over time. Beware of a whirlwind romance in problem solving.

PROBLEMS OF PERCEPTION.

Often a problem arises when someone has a faulty perception of you. They may underestimate you. This is not always a bad thing. They may negatively or positively generalise about 'people like you'. They fail to see you, they imagine a 'type' from central casting. They swiftly and stupidly categorise you in the type wardrobe that exits in their tiny brains and plonk the imagined you there.

This is something to be aware of. Sometimes their warped perception changes. It might not. The important thing to know is that you are not someone else's hallucination.

There are many other types of problems caused by perceptions. This book is full of them. Ask: is this a problem of perception?

PST 87: Perceptions govern brains - be aware of this.

Problems with people.

In order to get what you want you will have to interact with people in some way, even if over the Internet. There are many actions we can take to overcome problems with people:

Evade/hide/become invisible.
'Attack'/propagandise.
Accuse/resist.

Form alliances/divide opponents.
Compromise/negotiate.
Charm/assist.
Add value/remove pain.
Defuse/de-escalate through real or fake agreement.
Surprise/ambush.

Tactics are expressed through verbs. Change the verb, change the outcome.

PST 88: Most problems are people problems.

Dealing with types.

If you work out the 'type' a person self-identifies with you can often deal with them. People are predictable. Bureaucrats of all kinds operate a certain way: you need to know how to play 'em. You can work your way around the uptight stiff. Weirdos are best avoided. Or out weirded. The bore can be mollified by pretending you're fascinated. The narcissist can be ignored. The fanatic can never be reasoned with. The stick-in-the-mud can be left out. Remind the angry person of the importance of friends. The flake can go flake on his own. The control freak can be laughed at. The compulsive liar can be noted down as such. The goon can be fooled. The cunt will always be a cunt.

You'll work them out.

PST 89: Some people stereotype themselves. Their psychological strait jacket can be used against them.

Problems in connecting.

We live in weird times and weird times make people weirder. West World man is not evolving he is devolving. People, often of a sensitive nature, many times expect too much of others. These days people are quite fucked up but think they're normal. Rudeness has been normalised. Manners a relic of a bygone age. The social scene is increasingly hostile to normal interactions. Cultic 'thought' processes are widespread.

There are myths about connecting with others; one is the desirability of being a 'social butterfly'. These people generally come across as shallow. Then there is the desire to be 'promiscuous'; this fantasy prevents long-term bonding. It also puts an edge on all interactions reducing them to sex use value only. Not to mention that this is classic psychopathic behaviour engaged in by non-psychopaths.

Connecting genuinely. This can only occur when there is some 'natural spark' of connection. An ease almost from the get go. Do not seek quantity of 'friends' - the myth of 'being popular'. Seek genuine connectedness: this involves a shared sense of humour, being on the same wavelength and shared beliefs, differences are accepted and often found charming.

Do not seek the approval of strangers in such diseased times as these. Never try to impress anyone. Guys would do better with girls if they tried to impress them less. You are never going to get on with everyone. Who knows anyone with a thousand friends?

You can't hide your true self forever.

PST 90: Real connections occur when you're genuine.

Reinventing the wheel.

Sometimes problems are simply solved by new technology. However, on occasion people try to reinvent the wheel. There is no point. If there is a body of knowledge about how to solve problem X why not avail yourself of it? This is why we accumulate knowledge: to save time. Otherwise each generation has to start at step one.

I had a relative who wanted to make cider. He refused to try to follow any old recipes and procedures to start out. There is often a tried and tested **workflow** as we say in CGI (Computer Generated Imagery). Often solving any problem requires a workflow that works and leads to the desired objective. My relative failed to make one single decent pint of cider.

Step 1 - step 2 - step 3 = Solution state.

PST 91: On occasion you must step the beaten path first, then make your own paths.

Paradigm Shift.

There are times in life when things change forever. You can never go back to the old ways, the old 'system'. It has outlived its use perhaps. It was too destructive and an intervention occurs. Whatever.

Sometimes this is referred to as being on the right or wrong side of history. But even in our personal lives these shifts occur. We fall in love and get married. We have children. There is no going back. We have new problems, of a differing order. We must accept and adjust to them. A new job or role calls for new behaviours.

PST 92: Pointless problems occur when we struggle against the reality of reality.

How to excel at anything.

Talent + knowledge + practise + time.

There is a really simple formula to the problem of excelling at anything. You need natural talent. Your talents are resources. Then you need all the knowledge you can gather about that field: you should become a walking encyclopaedia. And you need practise. Theory is fine, you'll put it to the test and see what actually works. Practise is:

Effort + time + talent.

Practise is some kind of interactive magic between your efforts, failures, successes etc. It is the path to continued, consistent improvement. If you proceed in this manner with these simple principles in mind, at some point or another you will inevitably excel.

Everyone who is good at something gets better and better over time. Everyone has talents. Hone yours.

PST 93: If you improve your talents to the maximum you will achieve excellence. Something no one can take away from you.

Drawing red lines.

You must enforce your red lines aggressively. Many problems are caused by people being too patient in the face of provocation. But sometimes you must be patient - never let anyone provoke you to act until the time is right to act.

If I verbally draw a red line and let that person brazenly step over it - who am I really? People have to face the reality that sometimes problem solving requires sacrifice. Bullies in all guises understand one language - being 'smashed', one way or another. Brains baffle brawn.

PST 94: Red lines are your personal boundaries. 1 strike and you are out!

Tolerating the intolerable.

Good people put up with far too much shit from horrid people. Most of the world's woes come from good people tolerating the intolerable, putting up with a system run by ass/aresholes for arse/assholes. Your quality of life will be as good as you demand it to be. Every freedom ever won was fought for and taken from a tyrant. Nothing's changed.

PST 95: Sometimes nice has to turn to nasty.

Problems and control.

All problems confront you with the reality of control. How much leverage, influence, control etc. do you have over a situation? It will vary from 0-100%. This relates to ease of problem solving and how much resources, time, and effort you must allocate to achieve problem resolution.

Problem + degree of control = solution state.

Be 100% realistic in you estimation.

PST 96: How much control do you really have?

Bugs Bunny/Br'er Rabbit.

In life battles are often won by outwitting a dim opponent. There are many tales throughout history and folk-tale of superior wits deciding the day. You had better believe it. The English had an old saying, 'Tis better to fleece the Devil than fight him'. Keep you wits about you. Out think, trick an opponent if you must. It's okay to shit on arse/assholes. Use deception on the nasties. It's all enormously satisfying.

PST 97: Brains win the day.

To compromise?

You can't always get exactly what you want right now. What if you could get 50% of what you want? That is a forward moving achievement. Think of taking territory: at first you make your presence felt. Then you gradually go on to take more and more land etc. Make small achievements, and build from them. That's doable.

Compromise in the short-term: but always aim for 100% of what you truly want.

PST 98: Compromise on the path to getting what you want.

To push or not?

Do not make your move till you are ready. There is season for everything. Bide your time, when you are ready, and the time is right, then make your move. There is a time to push, to apply specific pressure. Often you must create the reason/excuse to make the push. Sometimes you wait like a fisherman - when the fish bites, you reel that sucker in. Trust your instincts.

PST 99: There is a time to apply just the right pressure.

Do not wait till things are perfect to act.

A good plan executed now is more likely to yield results than waiting for everything to be 'perfect'. Life is a compromise with reality.

Sometimes you wait till the time is reasonably good to act, not perfect. You may have to wait until a situation which broadly favours the execution of your plan comes into existence. This requires patience and long-term planning. The dice are not 100% what you want but they're good. When the time is the best it can be expected to be - strike. Act with resolve. This was US General Paton's dictum.

PST 100: A good plan enacted now is better than waiting for the perfect plan.

'Weight' loss?

You want to lose weight? Easy. chop off your arm. DON'T! What you want is to lose a certain amount of fat. You want to keep muscle and bone etc. Fat is not removed by varying types of starvation called 'diets'. Fat 'melting' occurs as a response to a good cardio-aerobic (heart-lungs) exercise routine that is 'low impact' - easy on your joints, muscles etc.

Moving your arms and legs in some sort of organised, rhythmic pattern in about 30 seconds bouts makes fat melt away. This is cardio magic. Even if you have 'emotional' problems around food. Perhaps it calms you. You'll feel a lot calmer when you exercise regularly. 2-3 days a week will do.

For fat loss in a sensible, doable way I recommend the excellent

YouTube channel Body Project (enter this or Body Project workout videos) - visit their website teambodyproject.com. If you go and do their beginner, low impact, fully standing YouTube workouts you will burn off fat fast, in a fun, positive atmosphere, with instructors who actually know what they're doing. Get ready for compliments. Their Youtube sessions are 100% free. I have no connections to this company. Thank me later...

Hitting the gym will give you muscles - fine if that's your goal. Specific problems require specific solutions. You can do all funky cardio workouts at home, in private for free. Soon you'll be able to design your own workouts. Problem solved.

When you reach your healthy goal shape - you change to a maintenance routine. You can be too thin - ladies, there is nothing wrong with being curvy. Guys - do cardio if you need to. It doesn't make you less masculine - it's actually fun and challenging.

Eat a healthy diet with all the food groups. Avoid too much sugar. But don't exorcise it from your life like a cheating lover! I love ice cream. Make sure fat makes up part of your food intake. You need some fat.

PST 101: Lose fat through aerobic-cardio workouts. Problems need solutions that work, that are safe, healthy, and have long-standing benefits.

A FAILURE TO ADJUST TO THE PERSON/ CIRCUMSTANCE.

Some people are the same with everyone. But there are ways to speak to different type of people. People with low intelligence must be handled in a certain way. The 'bureaucrat' requires a particular treatment - it is trained to follow formulas/patterns that it undeviatingly sticks to. Such creatures are easy to knock off balance by acting off script. Often the aim is to minimise tension or the escalation of a problem. Some people have to be played subtly. Notice the responses you're getting.

In the same way you may have to recognise the situation you are in. It may not be what you want, but it is what it is. Do as much as you can. But, a culture, a governing idea, cannot be ignored. Ideas, dumb or dangerous as they may be, are as real as brick walls. Sometimes you work 'around' a problem. You can only push so far now. You apply the 'pressure' available to you now. Then you pull back. Check the situation in the future. Has it altered? Can you do more?

What is the current reality facing you? Take this on board. Flexibility is a resource.

PST 102: Adjust to person and situation.

Circular problem solving.

Problems are not necessarily solved in a straight line. Take writing a book. You might get the idea for an ending first. You might have some powerful image from which the rest of the plot and story grow. You might come up with some dialogue that you want to fit in somewhere.

Problems can be fixed in this 'circular' kind of way. Problem solving often happens in a non-straight-line kinda way.

PST 103: There are linear and circular ways to solve problems.

Problem solving in the Age of Destruction.

The West is in a process of de-civilising. Destruction is spreading, like a cancer, looking for remaining healthy cells to devour. There is a war on for the very soul of the West. Everyday problem solving will continue much as before. However, one must be prepared for possible extreme disruptions in day to day living; think Murphy's Law. The prepared will thrive.

Both psychological independence and as much resource independence will help you get through such times. The post-World War 2 order is in free-fall. The centre cannot hold. A new order will be built. It must be built by the sane.

PST 104: Murphy's Law is the governing principle during crisis. But life continues...

Serving the masters of evil = fail!

If your problem is that the world should be a more nasty place I have a warning from history for you: you will fail, you losers always fail. If you take this knowledge to harm anyone good, you will unleash forces that you cannot even comprehend. If you serve the masters of evil your fate is sealed.

You have been warned.

PST 105: Your morality defines you and determines your fate.

'War'.

War may be said to exist when a state of affairs has been reached in which compromise and negotiations are no longer possible. The two sides are irreconcilably opposed. A 'fight' to prove the actual power relations between usually two sides ensues.

This may be a legal fight - so-called 'lawfare'. It may include the use of violence. As in an armed robbery etc. It may involve actual warfare between nation states/empires etc.

It may include a breaking off of all relations and an away from separatist movement where like minded people may mingle with each others without fear of 'other' imposed 'molestations' or violation of values.

When two sides cannot reach a civil agreement a 'war' of some kind is the consequence. A great deal of bluff and posturing will be employed. Deceptive tactics are absolutely essential in a war state. Available resources must be hurled energetically, intelligently, creatively but these must not be exhausted.

PST 106: War is inevitable when people will not compromise.

Making sacrifices for others.

In such Me-Me times the concept of sacrificing for others is totally alien. Yet at pivotal points in history sacrifice has turned the tide. There is a time to pivot. We are in a pivot time. Perhaps the most important yet. A sacrifice may not mean a loss of life. Old ideas and connections must sometimes be sacrificed.

PST 107: Sacrifice is sometimes essential.

The Old Knight and the Castle.

Once upon a time there was an old knight. He had been in the wars and wanted a castle to settle down in. As he rode through the silent forest he saw a great stone castle on a broad plain ahead of him.

He dismounted his horse and looked up at the old, grim fort. It looked just the ticket - he took a fancy that inside was something very special. It seemed unoccupied.

He tried to barge the door down. He tried to scale the walls. He tried digging under the castle. Nothing worked. He sat down and sighed. As he rested an idea popped into his head - "Build your own castle!" so that is what he did. If this were an ordinary tale that would be the end of the story.

A year and a day later he awoke from a weird dream. He stole out of the castle with a candle. All his servants were asleep. He went to the castle that could not be entered and pushed the massive wooden door. It opened and he stepped inside. It was full of cobwebs, broken things here and there. A most uninviting place...

PST 108: Appearances can be deceiving and...

EVERYTHING GETS SOLVED.

One way or another everything gets solved. I have never had a problem that didn't get solved in the end. Sometimes they just resolve themselves. Sometimes unexpected external factors come into play that change everything. Sometimes you 'outgrow' a problem. Something may happen that makes that old problem obsolete. A 'miracle' may occur. You may find a new source of info. You may learn from a new mentor. You may look at something in a new way. You may see a problem as a gift, an opportunity to develop.

Worry is great when it helps us - when it stops us taking stupid risks. It is bad when it paralyses our action. It is bad when it takes the joy out of life by making us constantly look out for danger. Sane worry works when it helps us anticipate problems that could arise. Never do anything that threatens your present and future prospects. Use your wisdom, it is a fact, not a faith, that one way or another you'll *solve that problem*, somehow, sometime, some way. We all do.

PST 109: Sooner or later all problems are solved.

Joining a cult won't solve anything.

Many people think that joining a 'cult' will allow them to solve all their problems. Cults have many faces. They possess no hidden wisdom. They won't, don't solve anything: they often do create a series of catastrophic problems that lead unsuspecting people to their doom. No one has all the answers. Life will never be perfect. There are no magic formulas. Joining a power-gang will not empower you; it will turn you into a slave. Stay away from cults.

PST 110: Cults create terrible problems. Keep out!

Out of your league.

Many people believe in a cultural myth - the idea of something being 'out of your league'. In a relationship context this often refers to a man or woman who is deemed so attractive that they are unapproachable by mere mortals and you shouldn't even try, or imagine they would ever be attracted to you. If you take this literally or as a general principle you would never aim to do anything above the lowest of ambition levels. We'd still be living in caves! What you want matters. You are a person of worth. You are a good person who loves and is loved. YOU deserve IT!

It is better to take on the idea that *nothing is out of your league*. You are worthy of any challenge if you have the ability and patience. With regards to looks, many people would be surprised what others find attractive in anyone. If you don't try at all you'll feel unfulfilled and regretful. Not something worth aiming for.

No one is 'better' than you. No one. People who imagine they are 'better' are the least important of all.

PST 111: You deserve what you want. Get it without apology. Enjoy your victory.

The problem of ageing.

Eat well. Sleep well. Exercise. If you exercise regularly you'll sleep well. Don't get sunburned too often if you're white, you'll end up like Otzi the Iceman. Over-exposure to the elements will age you.

Read and do the exercises from the book Eva Fraser's Facial Workout. I saw this lady on The Jonathan Ross Show in the 1990s in England. She was in her sixties but looked like a thirty-five year old. When I was 35 I started doing the face pulling secrets in her book. I am now 50 and look 28. The proof of the pudding is in the eating. I am also, I admit, vain.

Seriously though, bad people's bad thoughts engrave themselves on their faces as they age. Stress can be extremely ageing. Still your mind. We all age - whatever vintage you are, age well by taking care of yourself.

But most importantly - look after your teeth!

PST 112: Ageing does not have to mean crumbling.

A failure to observe.

Most people are unfortunately farts in trances. They wander around in a daze. Missing dangers and opportunities. Look at your average high street: 'Bring out your dead!' springs to mind. Look at the real world around you. Look at nature, architecture, people - really SEE people. Who are they really? What is the true nature of situation X, Y, and Z?

If you cannot observe reality accurately you will enter a doomed wrestling match. Reality always wins in the end. What is reality? Do you really know?

PST 113: Observe what is so. Then you'll solve things.

Families stick together.

If families only helped each other out more, especially during hard times. If someone in your fam is toxic then forget this. But if uncle John or auntie Jane just lost her job through no fault of their own - you can put them up on the couch rather than letting them become homeless. A strong, loyal, supportive extended family can survive any crisis, and problem - if it really does *pull together*. The most powerful unit in history is the family. With a united family all things are possible. Help family members who are down on their luck; if only selfishly - one day that could be you on the couch.

Look at royalty. They stick up for each other even when they commit crimes! They have each other's back. The common folk chuck their kids out at 18 and say sink or swim. Teach responsibility - don't teach turn your back.

PST 114: The family is THE problem solving force of the Ages.

Make opponents underestimate you.

You can often win by making someone underestimate you and overestimate themselves. Let them indulge in their faux superior image. When the time is right, at your choosing, reveal your true power. This will take them by complete surprise and stun them.

Act timid, weak and feeble - then figuratively grab their balls and yank up! Hard.

PST 115: Sometimes it is your advantage that opponents imagine you weaker than you are.

Laughter - your secret weapon.

The best medicine is laughter so they say. On this occasion they are right. Do you have a friend who always makes you laugh? Spend more time with them. Go get a laughter boost. People get too stressed too often when they forget to stop and see the funny side of things. Sometimes I think life is one, weird, big, absurd joke. And the joke is on me!

People in vastly worse dire straits than you have used humour to get through. And they did get through. Whenever something bad happens my dad doesn't get angry he laughs in such a way as to say - another fucking thing gone tits up! Life often has its tits up moments.

Making others laugh can help, and solve a number of problems. Your sense of humour is a resource. Use it. There is great strength in fun. More than you know. Never underestimate the power of ridicule - it is the giant killer. The contemporary comedian bullies the weak. Humour has always helped shrink egos.

PST 116: Laughter has explosive power.

Enjoy your own company.

Some people's biggest problem is being alone. They hate their own company. They are 'other' junkies. They constantly have to be around others. If they're not the anxiety builds and builds. STOP! What's so bad about you? Your breathe smells, you fart too much, scratch your butt in public but apart from that?

If you don't like being alone it's probably coz you are not busy enough. If you are focused on something absorbing you can spend hours happily occupied with it. You ever heard that saying you can be in a room full of people and still be lonely? It's true. If you *like yourself*, you are never lonely.

Of course we all need good company, but you need any or bad company like a hole in the head. It's okay to be on your own for a while. You won't die. Your head won't explode. The pixies really won't start talking to you.

There are times when you need a good 'ol thinking gumble anyway. Read a book, do something you want to do. Go for a stroll - look at all that beauty. People surrounded by beauty are never alone. How can you *like yourself* if you never spend any time with yourself?

PST 117: Spend time on your own to think, recharge your batteries, commune with yourself, reflect - get things done.

Ego - the big obstacle.

Every New Year, well, just after usually, as I go for my jog I see that sad creature - the New Year's resolution jogger. Sometimes he looks like he just woke up. Sometimes he has all the gear. He sees me and starts to have a race with me. He will defeat me - first time he's run in 30 years but. Then all of a sudden, after that vainglorious burst of manly effort, the reality of his abused body kicks in. He begins to look pained. He slows down. He's out of breath. I just carry on. He thinks I have defeated him. I was never in his imaginary race.

Oh the ego, usually male, but women can have their own conceited little egos. Never do something to please your ego. Your ego is a bit dumb. He can get you injured in a gym. He thinks his shit don't smell - till the fucker falls over backward in it. Psychopaths are all ego. Now you need a bit of ego: it gives you confidence and charm. Keep it on a leash. It's a tool, it is not the totality of you.

PST 118: Your ego can create big problems if you don't rein it in.

Evolution versus Revolution.

Change occurs in one of two ways - gradually over time or through a sudden, radical shake-up, usually during and following a crisis.

Knowing this the problem solver is armed with the knowledge that his or her strategies may take time to gain traction. The effect may be slow and plodding but noticeably progressive. It can be a powerful way of effecting change as it sneaks up on other people and has the effect of trapping them in a miasma of widespread change, perhaps over generations.

All revolutions are planned. Though they seem to explode from nowhere in response to an often manufactured crisis, the 'revolutionaries' have been plotting and waiting for the time to strike.

Radical change is always more easily accepted during overwhelming social upheavals. These have included, historically: plagues, wars, a changing of governance, new religions/ideologies, changes in morals, changes in social structures, invasions.

Although they may arrive with a hard punch caused by the chaos of the moment they may peter out after the initial ardour cools.

Positive *change* can happen in radical ways that *change* your life for the better. You will make that happen. The consequences will ripple through your life.

Each and both methods may prove useful to the problem solver.

PST 119: Gradual or radical? The choice is yours.

The individual that makes the difference.

All social systems fear one thing: the determined individual. Individuals have caused lasting change in human-consciousness down through the Ages. Their effect is as staggering as it is wholly unquantifiable.

This fact is expressed most obviously in the persons destined to be founders of the great religions. It exits too at multiple levels - the individual who fights for justice over cause X, Y, and Z. Someone, somewhere is always making a difference. Are you? You can.

As an individual never doubt your power. You are more powerful than you can conceive. This is known.

PST 120: The individual makes all the difference.

When giving up is good.

I have failed! Say it! When you've said it - you can get over it and try something else. NLP myth - there's no such thing as failure! That statement is a failure!

Haven't you ever royally failed, fucked up, embarrassed yourself? If you haven't - by Jove sir - you've never lived! When I was at University I was coming home by train and I grabbed my bag from the top rack. Yank! I pulled that fucker and it exploded! My underwear landed on some man's head. All my toiletries landed on another man's face - one by one. Boink! Boink! Boink! And he just sat there getting hit one at a time by my bits and pieces. I died that day. I shrank up my own ass with embarrassment.

Now I write a funny story about it that makes me smile. Point is:

sometimes you need to know when to surrender.

PST 121: Sometimes giving up THAT is winning.

Retire?

Retirement = DEATH! Don't retire. Do anything. Work part time. Never sit on your ass and do nothing but watch TV and stare wistfully out of the window. I have seen a man die in 3 months after behaving thus. He was so happy at first. Talking to neighbours, tending his garden. And then…One day he was sitting at his window looking out with a vacant stare of doom. Next thing I know a hearse it taking him off. Didn't plan. Didn't think. Don't use it - you'll lose it. Use your brain, use your body. Prolonged sitting is bad - get up - be active.

If you retire from a job do not retire from life. How are you going to be active in 'retirement'? I am never fucking retiring - I ain't even started!

I have a friend, he just turned 50. You'd think he was 35 - he plays tennis, lifts weights, jogs. He is looking forward to retiring. Thinking about playing golf! Buyer beware. If you think that ageing happens as you reach some milestone year you are wrong. Everyone ages - its all about how you'll age. I have no less energy now than when I was 25. In many ways I'm fitter.

Ageing is socially constructed: it's like a conveyor belt. Don't pretend ageing isn't going to happen, but if you do the right things you'll be a lot more sprightly than you can possibly imagine.

There is evidence that teetotallers are much more likely to get Alzheimer's.

My dad retired about 5 years ago. He was so actively involved in his job, it was his life's work. I knew it was a mistake. He sat and watched TV all day! He never had any health problems his whole life. Within one year he had sciatica, high blood pressure, and couldn't walk so well as he did. Within 2 years he got cancer - which he beat by, as he told me, having a 'fuck you cancer' attitude.

Now he works part time at his old job. He looks much fitter and happier. If you give up on life it will give up on you. We only get to go on this merry-go-round once - squeeze every moment out of life!

PST 122: Don't create problems by giving up on life or it will give up on you!

Do you really want to solve it?

Lots of people claim they want to solve problems. But they don't. Some want to talk about their problems - and then no nothing to solve them. Some people use certain problems to manipulate others. Some, perverse as it sounds, don't want to get 'better'. Some create new problems that merely add to the old and exacerbate them.

I used to ask clients with addiction problems on a scale of 0 - 10, 10 being totally committed, 0 being no desire at all, how much do you want to stop using X? It was rare to get anything above a 7. I had one or two 9s. I was the most motivated person in the room. No good.

I ask you again: do you really want to 100% solve that problem? Does your *unconscious* want to *solve it* too?

PST 123: If you really, really want to solve that problem it's half-way to being solved already.

'Cures', treatments, magic pills, 'side affects'.

A doctor I once knew told me every drug has long-term side effects. Are there 'cures' that are worse than the original problem? Sometimes undoubtedly. A cure, a real one is something that helps you *get rid of that problem* in its entirety. The problem state is fully replaced by the solution state.

Modern, allopathic medicine treats symptoms, doctors are not taught cures. If you have a pain in your foot you can take pain killers or get blind drunk, it'll probably hurt less. You might get addicted to those pain killers. Drinking too much is bad for you. What if it's the fact that your shoes don't have a supporting arch? You have flat fleet. Getting the right shoes fixes that.

What if you have hay fever every summer. You take pills. Ah, the magic pill that solves everything. You could buy a Hepa filter air purifier - these literally suck tiny particles, including pollen out of the air. Hospitals use them. If I get a bit nose tingly in early summer I turn mine on. *Problem gone.* Some people swear by one teaspoon of local honey every day. Will it work? I have no idea, everyone's different.

Long-running conditions may have to be managed. But, either way it can pay in more ways than one to try something new. Innovate in problem solving.

PST 124: Are you innovative enough to solve problem X?

Cry. It's okay.

When you are upset crying can let out unpleasant emotions. You can cry it out and feel better after. Often that upsetting thought goes too - the crying wrings it out. If you're a man - go cry in private. Tears can be beautiful. It's okay to be sad at times - sadness is not depression. The trees in fall or autumn are not unduly upset; they are doing what must be done. 'There is a season - Turn! Turn! Turn!'

PST 125: Appropriate crying gets rid of stress. Do not fear it.

Take the initiative.

People born after the late 1990s onward have been trained to follow orders. This never works in problem solving. Outside of war top-down mechanisms for problem solving always fail the individual with their one-size fits-all approach.

You must *take the initiative* in all problem solving. You initiate moves that will resolve the problem. Be your own champion. You reach out. You organise. You plan. You make goals happen through concerted wise action. You apply the pressure required to effect positive change. No one's coming to change your nappy.

PST 126: Problem solvers take the initiative.

The problem of the 'media'.

One of the main things the 'system' does is totally waste your life time. Waiting in queues. In traffic jams. Going to shit schools that teach you shit. Government measures that create new, easily foreseeable and worse problems. Jobs that are soul-destroying and pointless. The media makes you think all such time wasting is normal. It isn't. There is nothing in society that is not planned by those who ruin/run it.

The media sells you all manner of perverse idols and demands you emulate them. You are never a pleasing thing to them as you are.

Who made the media 'priests'? Literally one who leads the cattle.

How much time do you spend watching/interacting with any media? Are you culturally passive? Are you culturally active - creating culture? You are yourself culture. Culture production in all senses of that word requires time. How much more time are you going to waste? You are never getting it back. DO SOMETHING! BE SOMEONE!

PST 127: Problems are created by wasting time following 'false idols'.

Do the right thing.

If your goals and problem solving exertions are targeted at increasing good and happiness, general well-being, and good-will good people will note this, consciously and unconsciously, and will try to help you in your efforts. I have witnessed this almost semi-magical thing happen again and again.

PST 128: Good people naturally attract allies. Nothing is more powerful than the moral high ground.

To cheat?

There are lots of socially acceptable forms of cheating. People cheat at sports. Some people like a rigged game. Whatever.

Obviously you shouldn't cheat. If you cheated you didn't win, you scammed, you conned, you deceived.

Let's say you have a poor man, he has a family and can't afford his fuel bills. He lost his job for no good reason. He finds a way to mess with his energy metre. He keeps his energy costs down. Will you report him? There is moral relativism and there is compassion.

What is 'justice'? Is anyone doing you any favours?

PST 129: Immoral cheating is bad.

Truth and spirit?

I am not going to give anyone spiritual advise although many have spiritual problems. All I can say is that love of truth and true spirit are linked. Fearlessly pursue truth and spirit will manifest. Stay the fuck away from occult shit.

Ask yourself: why do so many violently fear truth?

PST 130: Truth seeking solves problems.

Carry on regardless.

As you solve problem after problem you *become more and more confident* in your problem solving abilities. Some people will try to derail this. Life has its ups and downs. CARRY ON REGARDLESS. This is your life, you have but one. Live your life or your own terms. It is ultimately your life. Laugh or smile at your detractors. Sometimes you do have to tell then to FUCK OFF. You are a unique human. You will have the same problems we all face and ones that no one else never will. Regardless, if they can be solved: YOU will solve them ;)

PST 131: The relentless win.

Printed in Great Britain
by Amazon